Sometimes Pasta

Recipe Starter

for Love Your Diet Menus

K.J.R. Alexander

Introduction

Sometimes Pasta is to help boost food preparation for the menus and list of Foods to Eat and weekly Sometimes Foods in the Love Your Diet books *Calories & Real Foods* and *Light Fantastic*. Since cooking experience varies among dieters, preparations from boiling an egg to baking bread are included. The homemade recipes for foods such as bread, pasta, pizza, and tacos are part of the *truth and proof* of the diet in redefining dieting beyond Stone Age Paleo to include the rich grains and foods of the Agricultural Revolution. The real culprits are modern manufactured foods.

The *truth* is that these nutritious homemade favorites are not fattening because they do not have the ingredients that stifle metabolism. This does not mean indulgence in homemade cakes and cookies is not fattening as described in the books about starch and sugar addiction. It simply means they are without the added strarch fillers, chemicals, excess salt, sugar, and questionable fats of manufactured ready-to-eat convenience and restaurant foods that make modern eating so tricky.

The *proof* is that you weigh yourself as described in the diet books. The lack of weight gain will prove to you how homemade versions of these favorite foods are not fattening and can be eaten with generous servings, but within reason of course. Conversely, the ready-made and manufactured varieties will increase weight, often for days, even though returning to the diet. Truth and proof. You will then be able to read store labels and order restaurant foods with some defensive understanding.

Food not only satisfies hunger but body and mind, soul and spirit. This is why you need to have a close relationship with your food. You need to get your hands on your food in preparing and eating it. Food you prepare yourself is more deeply satisfying, whether peeling an avocado or making pasta. Importantly, when you prepare your own food, unlike heat and eat, you can control the ingredients, such as adding herbs and spices in place of too much salt. Cooking food yourself on top of the range vibrates basic instincts of the comfort of an ancient campfire. You can see and smell the food cooking and add seasonings you like.

You don't have to be a chef to prepare something to eat. All you need are the ingredients and your appetite. If you haven't cooked much, once you gain some experience with preparing your own food, you will realize how easy and satisfying it is. Most of the knack of cooking is simply having the ingredients on hand.

The homemade bread recipe is worth the effort. It is nutritious, satisfying, and does not cause weight gain because you are preparing it with your own ingredients, ingredients that can be metabolized. Of course, you do not have to bake your own bread. Other options are fresh bakery breads without heavy sugars and preservatives as described in the diet books.

At the most basic, get ready to wash and slice some fresh vegetables and fruit, cook a little meat on top of the range, add bread and a bottle of wine, and eat gourmet on a budget!

Recipes & Food Preparation

Abbreviations
C = cup
T = tablespoon
tsp = teaspoon
qt = quart
oz = ounce

Simple Food Preparation for Love Your Diet
The Love Your Diet Plan does not have a lot of cooking especially during the day when easy dairy, fruit, vegetables, and snacks such as nuts and dried fruit are eaten. For the most part, dinners are simple, requiring cooking a protein source in meat, fish, or poultry, a "heavy-duty carb" such as rice or potatoes, and steamed vegetables. Easy desserts are fruits or no-sugar-added prepared foods. However, the menus also provide for delicious favorite foods such as pasta, bread, and tacos. But they need to be homemade to prove the point. As explained in the *Introduction*, this collection provides sample recipes of the added favorite foods that can be eaten without weight gain because they are prepared with basic real ingredients without additives.

Shopping Tip
The bulk foods section of your supermarket or a natural foods cooperative provides big savings in foods such as natural grains, flour, honey, herbs, spices, dried fruit, nuts, seeds, beans, and pastas. The savings in herbs and spices are especially rewarding.

Cleanliness
This is the first requirement of cooking and preparing good food. Everything needs to be clean – the surfaces, utensils, food, and you. Keep your hands washed. Keep hair covered with hat, scarf, or headband when cooking big recipes such as spaghetti sauce and bread.

Cranberry or Lemon Water

Get natural organic concentrated cranberry juice. Add 2 T to ¼ cup to a large glass of good tap or bottled water. For stronger juice, sweeten with honey or raw sugar. Fresh squeezed lemon juice is also good to add to drinking water. The fresh juice adds a sparkle of vitamins and metabolizers.

LYD - Love Your Diet Yogurt

Mix to taste: 2 T to ¼ C artificially sweetened, fruit flavored lowfat yogurt (100 to 120 calories) with all natural plain lowfat yogurt (no added sugar). The new versions of natural Greek yogurts are especially creamy and tasty, just watch sugar content. Fresh raw fruit such as blueberries or sweet black cherries makes any yogurt a satisfying feast. Avoid heavily sweetened yogurt at 200 to 300 calories. Artificial sweeteners are used during the early dieting phase but are to be phased out after experience with natural sugars.

Boiled Eggs

To prevent rubbery boiled eggs, cover with water, bring to a boil, then turn off heat and let set to desired doneness: 5 minutes for soft boiled and 10 minutes for hard boiled. (For jumbo-sized eggs, increase set time to 10 minutes soft boiled and 20 minutes hard boiled.) To serve, peel, mash with butter and add dash of paprika (rich in Vitamin A), cayenne, or turmeric.

Meats. Fish, Poultry - Cooking

For easy quick meats, gently fry in olive oil on top of the range. You can also use water in place of all or some of the oil. Season with garlic and pepper or other preferred seasonings. Frozen fish battered fillets can be heated in a heavy skillet, rather than the oven, until hot and crispy, turning to each side with spatula. No oil needed as there is oil in batter. For the Cornish game hen, stuff with 1 C freezer rice you made, season with salt, pepper, garlic, and lemon or lime and roast in middle oven at 325 degrees for an hour (see package for times). Brining meats for tenderness and flavor is the current trend. See online instructions.

Vegetables – Preparing & Cooking

Wash and pare raw fresh vegetables such as broccoli, green beans, or summer squash. Place on vegetable steamer rack above water in saucepan. Cover with lid. Steam over simmering water until of desired doneness. To serve, add 1 to 2 T lowfat sour cream.

Salad Greens & Leafy Green Vegetables – Preparing

Wash greens thoroughly. Spin dry in salad spinner or let drain dry in colander in sink. (They can also be patted dry with paper towels.) To store in refrigerator (spinach, kale) place *dry* greens in plastic bag.

Salad lettuce: After spinning dry, place in bowl and cover with damp paper towel, then with plastic wrap (paper towel keeps moist and crisp but not wet). Washed greens can also be stored in salad spinner if there is enough room in refrigerator (unlikely).

Tofu & Avocado or Hummus Appetizer

For an especially filling healthy snack or before dinner, cube (or mash together) one avocado and 1 oz tofu. Add favorite low calorie oil and vinegar type dressing. Eat with fork or spread on slices of fresh bakery or homemade bread. Hummus also makes a nutritious before dinner appetizer with natural bread or toast.

Vegetable Stew with Bread & Wine

1 - 2 large cans whole tomatoes
3 - 4 potatoes
¼ - ½ head cabbage
1 - 2 carrots
Salt, pepper, marjoram to taste
1 - 2 stalks chopped celery
Options with other vegetables: spinach, bok choy, green beans, parsley, peas, etc.

Prepare
Wash, peel, and chop vegetables and place in 6 quart stewing kettle. (Leave cabbage in one piece.) Add canned tomatoes cut into pieces and water to cover (canned diced tomatoes are too firm to cook up properly and add flavor). Of course, peeled and pared fresh tomatoes can also be used.

Cook
Simmer a few hours, adding water as needed, until tender and flavorful. (The celery and cabbage adds much to flavor.) Add salt, pepper, marjoram or other herbs to taste. If experimenting, season only a small bowl at a time until certain of flavor.

Serve
Serve with generous pieces torn from loaves of fresh buttered bread such as no-preservatives Italian, French, rye, or pumpernickel. Dip fresh or oven toasted bread into the juice as you eat the stew. Enjoy along with a glass of dry red wine.

Hot Cereal

Oatmeal

1 serving
¼ C natural rolled oats
Water to cover
¼ C diced apple or other fruit
1 T raisins, optional
1 T chopped nuts – optional
1 - 2 tsp raw sugar, honey, or natural maple syrup
2 T powdered instant milk or ½ C lowfat milk

Prepare and Cook
Assemble all ingredients except milk in bowl and microwave for 2 minutes or until oatmeal is soft.
Serve
Add milk and serve. If using instant milk, add water if needed. (Adding milk after cooking cools cereal to eating temperature.)

Whole Grain Cereals

Fine Ground Whole Grains
Prepare and Cook
Grain ground to fine granules will cook up as a "mush." Mix as above for oatmeal. Microwave 1 minute or until of desired doneness. Experiment and start with short cooking times as overcooking will make it rubbery.
Serve
Serve with milk and raw sugar or honey.

Chopped Whole Grains Cereal
Prepare and Cook
Assemble cereal and sweetener such as honey or demerara sugar. Cover cereal with water in small saucepan on stove. Simmer 20 to 30 minutes until soft. Or microwave 10 to 15 minutes or until soft. Add fruit (raisins, chopped apple) the last few minutes.
Serve
Drain any excess water and serve with milk and honey.

White & Wild Rice
(Wild rice adds rich nutrition.)

Small Recipe

(1 qt saucepan w/lid)
¾ C white rice - regular, jasmine, or basmati
1 C water approx. see first knuckle rule below
½ tsp olive oil
¼ C wild rice
1-2 T raisins
1-2 T sliced almonds
1-3 sliced fresh mushrooms

Large Recipe
for freezing in portions

(6 qt saucepan w/lid)
3 C white rice- regular, jasmine, or basmati
4 C water approx. see first knuckle rule below
1-2 tsp olive oil
1 C wild rice
½ C raisins
¼ C sliced almonds
½ C sliced fresh mushrooms

Cook White and Wild Rice separately due to different cooking times.

Cook Wild Rice
Rinse in water and drain. Cover with water in small saucepan. Bring to boil and turn down to simmer. Cook 40 minutes or until soft and chewy, adding water as needed. When done, drain excess water.

Cook White Rice
Rinse and drain rice 2 times. Add water and oil. Ratio is generally 4 parts water to 3 parts rice. First knuckle rule: measure water to the first knuckle of forefinger with finger sitting on top the rice. Stir briefly to mix. Bring rice and water mixture to boil. Boil gently one minute. Reduce heat to low simmer and cover with lid. Simmer 10 minutes (varies with type of rice, set timer and check) just until water is absorbed and rice is soft (but before rice is mushy and sticks to pan).

Mix White & Wild Rice and add other ingredients
Toss lightly together to mix: rice, wild rice, raisins, almonds, mushrooms.

Serve
Serve with dash of mild tamari soy sauce or butter. Add salt and pepper if needed.

Substitutions
Use brown rice in place of white rice and cook 40 minutes or until done.

Freeze
Scoop 1 cup servings into *foldover* sandwich bags (so you will have no air pockets). Shape oblong in bottom of bag and twist bag closed around rice to reduce air, *but without mashing or crushing rice*, and secure underneath. Place these 1 cup portions together into a larger freezer bag and freeze.
Yield: Small Recipe 4 to 5 cups. Large Recipe 12 to 15 generous cups. This freezer rice is ready in a moment to round out a meal.

Serve Freezer Rice
Take from freezer and remove frozen rice from plastic bag. Place in bowl and microwave 2 minutes or until thawed and hot. Serve with seasonings of choice or soy sauce.

Note: Without the mushrooms, this rice also makes a very nice breakfast cereal with fruit, raw sugar, and milk. Another reason why seasoning is best left for when served.

Rachele's Stir Fry

1 - 2 chicken breasts or thighs, boneless, skinless
2 T plus 1 tsp sesame or canola oil
2 T tamari soy sauce (low sodium tastes best)
2 cloves chopped garlic
1 C white basmati rice
2 C mixed fresh vegetables of choice, washed and chopped into 1-inch pieces: bok choy, snow peas, mushrooms, broccoli, cauliflower, baby corn, water chestnuts, red or green pepper, bamboo shoots, etc.
Spicy hot sesame oil to taste, optional
Black pepper to taste

Marinate Chicken
Slice into thin strips. Marinate in 2 T tamari soy sauce, 1 tsp sesame oil and 1 clove chopped garlic between 10 minutes and 1 hour.
Rice
Rinse rice in water and drain. Place in 1 qt. saucepan and cover with water up to first knuckle of forefinger resting on top of rice. Bring to boil and reduce heat to low. Cover with lid and simmer for 12-14 minutes (set timer). Remove from heat, fluff with fork, cover and let rest for 5-10 minutes.
Chicken
Heat skillet on medium heat with 1 T sesame or canola oil, add chicken and cook until almost done (2-3 min). Remove chicken from skillet and keep warm.
Vegetables
Heat 1 T sesame or canola oil, add washed and chopped vegetables to skillet and cook for a few minutes until crisp tender. Add 1 clove chopped garlic, return chicken to pan and cook together with vegetables 1 - 2 more minutes, until chicken is cooked.
Serve
Add rice to plate and top with chicken and vegetable mixture. Add tamari soy sauce, spicy sesame oil and black pepper to taste. Serves one to two. For four, double recipe. Leftovers nice for next day's lunch.

Tempura Battered Fried Vegetables or Shrimp

Ingredients
One package of dry tempura batter mix (available at supermarket)
Vegetable tempura: choice of raw sliced onion rings, mushrooms, zucchini
Shrimp tempura: *raw* fresh or thawed frozen, shelled, deveined shrimp (No tiny shrimp. Bigger is better: minimum 20 to 30 count)
1/2 cup olive oil for frying (enough to cover bottom of skillet and cook one side of the food at a time)
Chopped fresh garlic (optional)

Prepare vegetables
Wash and slice vegetables.

Prepare shrimp
Shell if needed, wash, and check shrimp that vein along back is removed. Drain on paper towel or pat dry. Place some of the dry tempura mix in a plastic bag. Add shrimp and shake in bag, coating shrimp with dry mix before dipping in tempura batter.

Prepare batter
Mix water with tempura mix in a bowl as directed on package or to desired thickness and set aside. Thinner batter cooks up lighter and fluffier. Experiment. The batter will get thicker as it sets. Add chopped garlic to batter.

Cook
Heat olive oil in skillet. Test readiness by cooking one piece. Dip vegetables or shrimp in tempura batter and then fry, turning to each side. Drain on plate with paper towel.

Serving suggestions
Serve shrimp with lemon wedges and cocktail sauce, rice, and white wine. The onion rings are nice with the shrimp or alone as a lunch or afternoon snack with red wine.

Fish Cakes

1 - 15 oz can **red salmon** or mackerel
1 egg
1 C rolled oats (*thin-cut* oats) or corn meal or cracker crumbs
1/4 C olive oil

Mix and shape
In bowl, mix fish with egg by stirring with fork. Put oatmeal on a plate. With hands, shape fish and egg mixture into 3 to 4 patties. Put patties on plate of oatmeal and coat both sides by turning and pressing.

Cook
Heat olive oil in skillet. Add fish cakes and fry until golden brown on outside and hot on inside. (No salt is needed as the canned fish already has salt.)

Serve
Serve hot with lemon wedges, soy sauce, or tartar sauce.

Store
Leftovers can be stored in refrigerator for heating in microwave next day.

Tacos

1-2 dozen yellow corn tortillas
1-2 pounds lean hamburger
1 C tomatoes, fresh, diced
1 C grated cheese
2 C lettuce, spinach leaves, or mustard greens, shredded
Chopped fresh garlic to flavor
Salt & pepper
Cumin, powdered or seeds to flavor
1/3 C cold-pressed olive oil or corn oil
Taco sauce or salsa
Sour cream

Prepare
Tomatoes, lettuce, cheese.

Cook Hamburger
Place hamburger in skillet to fry, adding garlic and cumin, pepper, and light sprinkling of salt. Fry hamburger in own juices or, if very lean, add water or oil. Set aside.

Cook Tacos
Heat olive or corn oil in another skillet to cook tortillas. (Cover bottom of skillet with oil and turn tortillas to cook other side.) When hot, place each tortilla in oil quickly to soften, first one side, then the other. Turn with long fork and metal spatula in each hand or use tongs. Turn carefully to prevent tearing and to prevent hot oil from splashing. Fold in half and cook longer for crisper tortillas. Experiment as to preference. Drain on paper towels on plate.

Assemble and Serve
Add hamburger, tomato, cheese, taco sauce, sour cream, and lettuce to the middle of each tortilla, fold over sides and eat with hands using paper napkin (tacos deliciously oily).

Store
Fully assemble tacos and place each in fold-over sandwich bag or plastic wrap and refrigerate. To eat, heat for 8 seconds or until of desired warmth in microwave.

Rice & Bean Burritos

8 - 10 large flour tortillas
1 lb black beans or pinto beans or both mixed, ½ lb each
2-3 large ham hocks
1 C white or brown rice, rinsed 2X
1 C grated cheese
1 C lowfat sour cream
Salt, pepper to taste

Prepare and Cook
Cook hamhocks and beans day before or earlier in day.
Wash, cover with water, and simmer hamhocks for a few hours until tender.
Rinse beans 2-3 times. Add to ham hocks in water to cover. Simmer several hours adding water as needed until beans are soft.

Add rice to beans and bean soup and simmer until rice is done and absorbs bean liquid (white rice, 10 to 15 minutes; brown rice, 40 minutes, see package directions). Season with salt and pepper.

Serve
Heat tortilla for a few seconds in microwave to soften. Fill tortilla with bean and rice mixture and top with grated cheese and generous sour cream. Roll and fold over to form burrito and eat.

Store
Place ingredients in refrigerator to assemble and heat. To freeze: wrap each assembled burrito in tin foil.

Krista's Pasta Sauce

4 - 6 medium, sliced zucchinis
1 C sliced mushrooms
½ C chopped onions
1 T olive oil
½ lb ground turkey
4 cloves fresh garlic, chopped
1 large can of tomato sauce or large jar organic marinara sauce
Oregano
Basil
Garlic powder
Salt and pepper
Dash cayenne, optional

Prepare
Zucchini, mushrooms, 2 garlic loves, onions.

Sauté
Zucchini, mushrooms, 2 garlic cloves, and onions together for 5 minutes. Let simmer on low heat in small amount of olive oil or water.

Cook turkey In a separate pan
Add olive oil and turkey and sprinkle with pinches of oregano and basil, salt and pepper, the 2 remaining cloves of garlic, and garlic powder. Cook for five minutes, sautéing.

Put the two mixtures together
Cook together on low/medium heat for 10 minutes, stirring occasionally. Season to taste with more oregano, basil, garlic, and dash of optional cayenne.

Serve over durum whole wheat pasta of choice, cooked to package directions. Servings: 3-4.

Pasta Dinner

¼ lb. regular fettuccine
5 - 10 pieces spinach fettuccine
2 - 4 T olive oil
¼ C chopped garlic
½ C sliced mushrooms
4 - 6 fresh raw spinach leaves
2 T grated parmesan cheese
1 loaf soft French or Italian bread, split, spread with butter, olive oil, and chopped raw garlic

Cook
Add fettuccine to 3 quarts boiling water and cook until soft and easily cut with fork. Drain in colander. Heat olive oil in skillet (large enough to hold pasta, added later). Cook mushrooms and spinach leaves in oil. Turn off heat and add chopped garlic. Stir in fettuccine.

Serve
Top with parmesan cheese and serve with heated or unheated garlic bread, fresh salad, and chianti or other red table wine.

Store
Place covered leftovers in refrigerator. Heat in microwave to eat.

Variations
Substitute other pastas such as linguini in place of regular fettuccine. In place of olive oil and vegetables, make tomato sauce or buy prepared sauce made with natural ingredients. Read labels. Be creative and use ingredients you prefer.

Meat & Mushroom Tomato Sauce for Pasta

1 medium onion, diced
¼ C olive oil
½ green pepper, chopped (optional)
2 cloves garlic, chopped
1 large can tomato sauce
Salt to taste (canned tomato sauce also has salt so no additional may be needed)
Pepper to taste
Granulated garlic to taste
Oregano to taste (the primary characteristic taste for Italian flavor.)
Optional to include: sage, basil, rosemary, thyme)
½ C sliced mushrooms
1 lb. ground mild Italian sausage

Cook
Sauté onion on low heat in olive oil until soft and transparent but not browned or carmelized. Add tomato sauce. Add ¼ can water for cooking down. Add green pepper, mushroom, and chopped garlic and simmer at least 30 minutes or until sauce cooks down. Add granulated garlic, salt, pepper to taste, some of herbs. Add more herbs after sauce is cooked to preserve flavor: turn off heat, add herbs, cover and let stand.

Meatballs
Use 1 pound of ground mild Italian sausage and gently shape into meatballs. Simmer in skillet with water covering bottom of pan (in place of oil). When done, add meatballs only, without fatty drippings, to sauce.

Serve
Spoon sauce and meatballs over pasta.

Store
Excess sauce can be refrigerated for a day or frozen.

Mike's Grilled Steak

T-bone or New York Steak, 1 per person
Montreal Steak seasoning
Garlic powder
Onion powder
Salt & pepper

Season Steak
Take steak out and scrape off any dust from being cut. Sprinkle both sides with a little Montreal seasoning, a little onion powder and a little garlic powder. Add touch of salt and pepper. A little of all these go a long way. Rub in spices on both sides.

Cook on Ready Gas Grill
Sear on high for 4 to 5 minutes, turn over and do the same. Then turn 90 degrees and over and go 4 to 5 minutes on each side, depending on thickness.

Serve
Let rest on plate for 5 to 7 minutes before cutting.

Option: Cook on Top of Stove in Skillet
Season as above and cook with 1 T olive oil. Sear on both sides in moderately hot skillet. Turn off heat or set to low and cover. Let set until of desired doneness. Rare, just a few minutes. Medium well, about 15 minutes. Test by cutting into steak and checking redness or best, use meat thermometer.

Lobster Tail from Frozen

Purchase and Thaw
Buy cold water lobster tails which are of better quality than those from warm water. (If small, get 2 per person if within budget.) Thaw in refrigerator 8 to 10 hours before cooking.

Cook
Bring a large pan of water to boil and drop lobster in. Cook one minute for each ounce of lobster.

Serve
Drain and serve with clarified butter and lemon. You can also simply use melted butter in place of the clarified. Check online for additional ways to prepare lobster.

Clarified Butter
Heat 1 cube (2x the amount of clarified butter you need) unsalted butter in pan on stove. Heat on low heat until milk particles turn a light brown and settle to bottom of pan. The foam on top is the milk whey which you can skim off with a spoon. Process takes about 30 minutes of very low heat. Check frequently. If overcooked, the milk at the bottom gets too brown (then it is called butter ghee). Drain off the clarified butter oil into a serving dish. Also, there are excellent online instructions for clarifying butter.

Bread Recipes by Love Your Diet

Recommended is to get a bread machine and make your own bread with little effort. That way, you know what is in your bread. A bread machine also stirs and whips the dough to stretchiness, replacing hand kneading or multiple risings. Panasonic is a good reliable heavy-duty machine. A new machine is best as it comes with instructions. Bread machines are also common at garage sales and thrift shops but you will need to get online recipes and experiment more, as instructions and recipes are not usually included. Used machines may also have scratched coating in bread pan.

Of course, you should not make the bread recipes that are packed with refined white sugar. Your own homemade whole wheat bread (or half wheat and half white flour) is delicious and **not fattening**! You'll be amazed at how you much of this satisfying bread you can eat and not gain weight. You can experiment with morning weigh-ins as your proof.

However, there is also a question as to the teflon coating on cookware and teflon lines the bread machine basket. Manufacturers claim that very high temperatures (around 600 degrees) have to occur before the chemical is released. If this is a question for you, you can mix the bread in the machine and then bake it in the oven.

Recipes for making the bread without, then with, a bread machine are given below. Use a bread recipe you like as your standard bread so you will know the recipe, be able to maintain consistency, and easily make a loaf of bread anytime.

Whole Wheat Bread
1 Large Loaf
Without Bread Machine

1½ C all-natural stone ground whole wheat flour (Bob's Red Mill is good)
1½ C unbleached white flour
1½ tsp salt
1 tsp wheat germ – optional
1 tsp wheat bran – optional
1½ C lowfat lukewarm milk*
2 T demerara sugar or raw honey or combination
3 T cold press olive oil or natural salted butter or combination
1½ tsp dry, fast-acting, or bread machine yeast

*The balance of milk to flour depends on the consistency of the flour used. For example, whole wheat flour may absorb more liquid than white flour. Also, using honey rather than sugar can affect how much moisture is needed. See recipe below for adjustments.

Prepare pan
Prepare loaf pan, approximately 5" x 9", by liberally buttering bottom, sides, and top edge. Use crumpled paper towel to spread butter. The best type of pan is tinted glass as tinted glass browns bread more readily and the see-through glass allows checking for browning. (Follow pan instructions for safe handling of glass baking containers.)

Prepare dry ingredients
In medium-sized bowl, add flour, salt, wheat germ, wheat bran. Mix briefly with spatula or large spoon. (This sticky-dough bowl can later be cleaned with water and a throw-away paper towel.)

Prepare wet ingredients and yeast
In separate bowl or measuring cup, add milk, then yeast to dissolve, sugar, and then oil. The milk needs to be lukewarm to slightly warm to help activate the yeast, so warm 40 seconds in microwave if needed (but *without* yeast, as high microwave heat can "kill" the yeast). Stir all ingredients to blend. As indicated above, raw honey can replace the sugar or the two can be combined to make 2 tablespoons. Similarly, butter can replace the oil or be combined with oil to make 3 tablespoons. (The honey and oil help keep the bread soft and moist.)

Mix
Add milk mixture to flour mixture. Stir to mix. All flour should be moistened without any dry patches. If needed, add more milk, a tablespoon at a time, until dough is completely moistened. (Cold milk is okay here as it is not enough to cool the dough.) The surface should slightly glisten with moisture but not be wet and thin. If too much milk is added, sprinkle flour, no more than 1 tablespoon at a time, until right consistency. Avoid extremes: dry stiff dough will make dry bread; wet, loose dough will make thin loose bread. After mixing, let dough rest 3-5 minutes.

Rise #1
Butter clean hands liberally. Shape dough in bowl into a ball. Lift out, shape into loaf, and place in *loaf pan* (or place in pan and pat down). Cover loosely with plastic and let rise in a warm, draft-free place until double in bulk, about 1-2 hours. It is double in bulk if finger punched in dough retains the finger hole. (If you cannot lift dough from bowl because it is too loose, it is too wet. Add sprinkles of flour as above.)

Rise #2 (The second rising increases the stretchiness and flexibility of the bread.)
Butter hands liberally and punch down dough, pressing out air. Lift dough out of pan and shape into loaf, pressing out all air and rolling under for a minute (this is a mini-kneading). Place dough back in pan and let rise again, loosely covered as before, to double in bulk.

Bake

Bake in preheated 350° oven, on middle rack, for 30-35 minutes. Loaf should sound hollow when tapped lightly on top with finger and sides and bottom are browned. Remove from oven and butter top of loaf.

Cool

When bread is cool to touch, turn out of pan to cool at room temperature. When completely cool, place in plastic bag and refrigerate. Wipe out any condensed moisture with a paper towel or reverse plastic bag to get rid of moisture. When completely cooled in refrigerator, bread slices easily to desired thickness.

Store

Store bread in refrigerator to keep fresh for a week or more. To freeze for later use, wrap bread, still in plastic bag, with tin foil and date.

Two Loaves
Without Bread Machine

Double the recipe, use a larger bowl and 2 loaf pans. Here is the double recipe.

2¼ C whole wheat flour
2¼ C unbleached white flour
3 tsp salt
1 T wheat germ (optional)
1 T wheat bran (optional)
3 tsp dry, fast-acting, or bread machine yeast
1 ¾-2 C lowfat lukewarm milk
4 T demerara sugar or raw honey or combination
6 T cold press olive oil or natural salted butter or combination

Mix and Bake

Mix and let rise two times as above in the two loaf pans and bake.

Bread Machine 1 loaf

Mix dough as above for one loaf without bread machine. You need to mix the dough separately in a bowl before adding to the bread machine to be able to see and control the amount of moisture as in the hand-mix recipe above. After mixing to a slightly glistening dough, place dough in bread machine. Add the yeast separately to dispenser according to bread machine instructions. If no separate yeast dispenser, add yeast to milk mixture as in hand-mixed. Set to quick-bake at 3 hours in the bread machine.

Mix Dough in Bread Machine and Bake in Oven

1 loaf

Add dough and yeast as above for bread machine. Set machine to "dough." The machine will whip and mix the dough and let it rise. When timer sounds, remove dough from machine and with clean buttered hands, punch down and shape the dough into a loaf, place in buttered loaf pan, and let rise. After dough rises in pan to double in bulk, bake in oven at 350° for 30-35 minutes as above. When using the bread machine, you do not have to let the dough rise two times in the pan but just the once before baking.

2 loaves

The bread machine makes baking 2 loaves a breeze. Just use the double recipe for 2 loaves above, reserving the yeast for the dispenser. The bread machine is made to bake only 1 loaf. However, it can **mix** dough for 2 loaves. Also, you have to make sure the increased dough doesn't rise up and spill all over the machine. Therefore set to "dough" and time it for 1 hour or until the dough is whipped and has only just begun to rise near top of bread machine pan. (Open lid of machine and check. Since you are not baking in machine, it will not matter that you cool the temperature by opening the lid.) Then remove dough to two buttered loaf pans and let rise until doubled in bulk and bake at 350° for 30-35 minutes as above.

Pizza Dough from Bread Recipe

Each one loaf recipe makes two 10″ pizza crusts or one double-crust 10″ pizza. Use an oven-suitable skillet (no plastic handles that can melt) for the double crust pizza so you will have room for everything. Or, of course, you can make a square pizza in a square pan of comparable size.

To freeze pizza dough for later use

Each one pound loaf recipe makes two 10″ skillet-sized or one 10″ double crust pizza. Put dough in refrigerator and let cool until it stops rising. (Freezing with air bubbles ruins dough.) Then butter hands and squeeze air out of dough, forming into two balls. Place balls of dough in foldover sandwich bags and twist tightly to keep air out. Place in larger freezer bag such as zip lock or wrap in tin foil, label and date, and freeze.

Prepare to bake

Remove from freezer and let thaw until yeast starts acting and dough is soft and puffy. Stretch and flatten each ball into a layer as you build a single or double crust pizza of your choosing.
Ready to bake when dough starts to get a little puffy and soft again. See bake below.

Simple Pizza Sauce

Sauté slowly in saucepan 1 cup chopped onions in 2 tablespoons olive oil until soft and transparent (but not scorched or brown which will affect taste). Add 1 medium can tomato sauce (enough for two 10″ pizzas or one double crust) and 2 chopped garlic cloves. Add a little water and let simmer and cook down slowly until thickened. Add oregano only, or also basil, then salt, pepper, and garlic granules to taste. Top with favorite ingredients (olives, mushrooms, Italian sausage, Canadian bacon, pineapple) along with topping of grated mozzarella and parmesan cheese.

Bake at 350° for 20 min single, 40 to 60 min double until edges are brown and cheese is melted.

www.ingramcontent.com/pod-product-compliance
Lightning Source LLC
Chambersburg PA
CBHW061950280526
45787CB00004B/1798